# DRAMA IN THE OPERATING THEATER

WHAT HAPPENS IN THE OR WHEN THE PATIENT GOES TO SLEEP

DR. MURANO SERIES
BOOK 1

WITOLD NIESLUCHOWSKI

VERBA VOLANT,
SCRIPTA MANENT.

*To Bonnie's Parents who at the moment are going through the hard times*

# 1

## PROLOGUE

PROLOGUE

Just imagine . . .

After a thorough evaluation of what seemed like banal shoulder pain, you find out it's not so trivial. You need open-heart surgery. Your first thought is, *What have I done wrong?* Then comes acceptance and you decide to fight for your health. The cardiologist refers you to a surgeon he says is the best around.

The first step is to read all about your heart problem. The internet overflows with a deluge of data. Next come the conversations with your friends, seeking opinions about the surgeon. You meet him and ask questions. Then more questions. After a certain point, you realize all these questions aren't getting you anywhere. And you're still uneasy deciding who will operate on you. You're not satisfied. So, as many articles recommend, you look for a second opinion. The next surgeon sounds better and, after talking to your friends, you ask him to operate. Then comes another visit and more questions. Some of his answers differ from the ones given by the first surgeon. He smiles and tells you that, in essence, it doesn't matter. But you are still suspicious. *It's my heart he's going to cut*, you think. Finally, after being interrogated for an hour, he tells you that in the end, to operate, he must have your full confidence. Otherwise, he doesn't want to be your surgeon. You say you trust him and want him to be your doctor. The office secretary schedules the case.

IN THE PREP room before surgery, your brain is racing. *What's going to happen in the OR while I'm asleep?*

THE PROCEDURE IS OVER, and you slowly wake up. You see the surgeon coming into your cubicle in the recovery room. He smiles, asks how you're doing and how much pain you have. Not fully awake yet, you say, "Not that much, less than I expected." And then, "How did it go?"

He smiles again and says, "Fine, you did great, nothing out of the ordinary." But then he adds, "Nothing we couldn't handle."

Something shoots through your brain, and now you're completely awake. *What happened that he had to "handle"*?

*What really happened while I was unconscious on the operating table, defenseless, my heart exposed for all to see? Did they cut something important and then have to fix it? Was I seriously bleeding, did they struggle, and now they don't want to tell me?*

The truth is that cardiac surgeons are people like the rest of us. For this short time, while you are on the operating table, your life and his life run together. Your birthplaces, your upbringings, your life stories are most likely as different as doing surgery using the traditional open method or doing the same procedure through a scope. The ways and means are different, but the goal is the same. You both want to have the best possible outcome.

So, for several hours, your lifepaths ran together. Incredibly linked. If one believes the heart is a metaphor for life, the surgeon held your life in his hands. He was privileged to see the inside of your body, a view you'll never be privileged to experience and, frankly, no one else in your life will either. Not even your spouse. Your surgeon was in complete control of your fate, and you don't even know what he was doing. You assume, and pray, he's your best friend. Because whatever he does affects your future. It's like flying on a big 747, and he was the pilot. If something went terribly wrong and the plane went down, though, he wouldn't be hitting the ground with you.

Wouldn't you like to be a fly on the wall during surgery? Well, there are no flies in the operating room. At least there shouldn't be any. What about watching the procedure on a hidden camera? Not your incision, just his face. And hands. And his voice.

All kinds of things happen in an operating room. There are so many factors involved in surgical procedures. Countless people are involved in the care of the patient in the operating room alone: they invade the patient's body, administer potent medications, and use complicated machinery. All must go right for the surgeon, and the patient, to claim success. Surgeons have private lives: conflicts with spouses, children using drugs, parents getting sick and dying, and financial problems like the rest of us. Some of them drink alcohol, occasionally even more than they should. Some take drugs. Like in any workplace, there can be personal conflicts between the operating room staff. And when you close all these people within the four walls of an operating suite, fill the space with strong egos, and add the often quickly changing, dizzying events in the room, you have all the ingredients for a fast-paced action movie screenplay. Everyone has a different tolerance level for stress, and this can result in real drama. A script for a gripping, real-life story.

Is this is why the original name for the operating room was an operating theater?

# 2

# THE STORY

He was riding in the back of a car. It was an old model. There were no seat belts. He could hear the conversation in front.

"I can drive," the female voice said.

"I'm okay," the man said.

"You've been drinking. You swore you'd never drink and drive again."

"I said I'm okay. It wasn't that much. And, by the way, I told you not to flirt with that guy."

"I didn't. He was just being nice to me. You never are."

"I was pissed, dammit!" Jack heard the man yelling and hitting the steering wheel with both hands.

The car jerked and Jack swayed from one door to the other. Then, suddenly, he heard the woman's piercing voice.

"Look! Oh no!" she cried.

Jack looked over the front bench seat and saw the woman's hand outstretched towards the windshield, then her other hand pushing back in his direction. In a flash, he saw the headlights of the other vehicle hitting theirs. There was a terrible screeching noise, a flash of white light, and then Jack woke up.

HE COULDN'T BREATHE, couldn't move. He was covered in sweat; his heart was racing. He looked at the bedside clock. Big red numbers showed 4:21 a.m.

The day ahead would again be blighted.

It was a moment in time Jack could not escape. Not in thirty years. The screeching of the tires as the family car went crashing into the huge dump truck had drilled deep into his mind the remainder of his life. But what stayed with him above all else was his mother's ear-splitting, "Nooo!" while she reached her open hand to the back seat, as if trying to push her five-year-old son away from this horrible collision, a desperate effort to save him.

That was the last time Jack heard his mother's voice. Moments later, he vaguely recalled people frantically pulling his family out of their mangled Ford. His father's face was bleeding as he tried to assist the rescuers. His mother was silent. She did not move. Later, he found out they'd taken her to the morgue.

His mother's parents drove him to the funeral. The service was held at a small chapel located in the cemetery where she was to be buried. He remembered the sounds of people singing, a few speeches, and then they carried his mother's urn to the wall full of brass plaques. One of the compartments was open, and his grandpa put the urn inside. Then Jack watched as the old man stood there, praying.

When it was Jack's turn to approach the crypt and say goodbye to his mother, he looked up to his grandma and stretched out his hand. She opened her purse and gave him a toy. It was a small teddy bear, the last Christmas gift he had received from his mother. Jack took it, looked at his favorite toy for the last time—a moment longer than necessary—and then he placed it next to the urn in the small crypt. He'd seen the grown-ups praying, and he, too, tried to stand up with his hand on the crypt. He wasn't sure how to pray, so he just stood there, waiting for the tears to stop. He didn't want the other people to see him crying.

Then he remembered a couple of workers fixing the front marble plate to the wall now containing his mother's urn. It would take time, Grandma told him, to make the brass plate with Mom's name.

Those were Jack's memories of his mother's death and burial.

He looked at the bedside clock again. Five o'clock. Still at least an hour before he had to get up for his morning drive to the hospital. So, he just lay there, his hands under his head, staring up at the ceiling, with Diane sleeping quietly next to him. As always, he was careful not to wake her.

~

JACK DIDN'T WANT to do this surgery.

He knew the risks were high and the benefits minimal. He felt pressured again by the patient's cardiologist to take him to the operating room. Dr. Kaplan, the director of cardiology, had told Jack that there was nothing more he could do for this elderly, sick patient. As a medical doctor, Kaplan said, he had used all his tools. The patient was too sick. Mechanical problems with the valve and coronary arteries had to be treated by mechanical means, so surgery was the only way to go. Jack had this sinking feeling that the cardiologist just didn't want to be involved any more in the care of this extremely ill patient.

Mr. Holden's heart was as enlarged as it was weak––both bad signs. He needed to have his aortic valve replaced and three coronary arteries bypassed. The surgery itself could kill a younger man, but Victor's poor heart added to the risk exponentially. Were he to die after surgery, the family would be devastated and may even be angry, no matter how thoroughly Jack explained the risks. Jack would be crushed, and the cardiologist would be absolved of any responsibility. Still, Jack felt he had no choice, since he had refused Kaplan's previous case. Refusing this case could put this cardiologist referral channel at risk of drying out. So instead, he had to make every effort to present himself as a fighter for the patient's best care.

He would have to explain their patriarch's grave situation to Holden's family once again. He would assure them that he would do everything in his power to get Mr. Holden through this difficult surgery and make him well. He'd already told them that there would be bumps in the road, but as their family surgeon, he would be with them the entire way, and he would use his best skills and judgement in the operating room and during the recovery. He would repeat all that this morning in his conversation with Holden's family before the surgery.

Jack had another problem, though. In recent months, one of his patients had died and another was still on a ventilator and on dialysis after a protracted and complicated surgery. In his mind, malpractice lawsuits were looming. He knew he was being watched by the chief of staff, and any more complications in the OR could result in a warning from the executive committee, if not a suspension.

His reputation as a surgeon, his career—everything—was on the line. He had no choice but to take on this case. And in doing so, he felt himself on the verge of being crushed between the proverbial rock and a hard place.

FINALLY, Jack welcomed the bedside clock flashing 6:00 a.m.

He didn't have the time or the will to eat now––coffee and doughnuts in the doctors' lounge would have to do. Diane and the kids were still asleep. On his way out, Jack looked through the opening of the door to his son's bedroom and saw Mike's blond hair on his black pillow. The boy had designed the color scheme of the room himself. White walls, black sheets, and contemporary fixtures. Jack smiled, thinking about how his son's modern tastes clashed with his father's more traditional upbringing.

Driving toward the California 101 freeway, Jack didn't even notice the street traffic getting congested, signal lights slowing him down, or the other drivers cutting in front of him. He felt as if he were driving in a fog. Now the freeway became a blur. His mind drifted back to the day of the accident, the last day he saw his mother. Then to the last day he saw his father. That day also stayed with him forever.

But not only with him. Thirty years later, the day of his father's sentencing was still emblazoned in the minds of those in the community who had attended the trial.

THE COURTROOM WAS full that day. After a highly emotional, week-long trial, the members of this small Northern California town now awaited the sentencing. The crime had been committed a year ago, and Mr. Murano had lived in the community for ten years, ever since marrying a local girl. These people knew his little boy, Jack, who, after his mother's death and his father's incarceration, had been living with his grandparents. Both were in their seventies, sick, and unable to make the final court session that day.

The mahogany door opened and a bailiff entered the room. In a moment, the noisy hall became quiet. All eyes were directed to the officer of the court.

"Everybody rise," the bailiff said. His voice matched the power of his uniform. "Department 23 of Sutter County Court is now in session, with Judge Boleno presiding."

A black-robed woman appeared in the door, scanned the court, then decisively marched to the podium. Judge Boleno was a petite, gray-haired woman. She didn't look like a person who could take on hard criminals, cunning lawyers, and noisy crowds, but she was. She was known as a tough jurist, but at the same time, she was a compassionate person whose many years on the bench had earned her the respect of the community. She sat down, almost disappearing in her massive black leather chair. Behind her, on the wall, were flags of the United States and California, with the Seal of Sutter County hanging well above her head.

"Please be seated," she said.

After a subtle rustle as people sat down, Judge Boleno's court became quiet again.

"I want to open the proceedings for the sentencing hearing of John Murano," she said, opening a large black folder and pulling out a document. The judge then raised her head.

To her right, behind the table, she saw the defendant in a bright orange jumpsuit, with an attorney on each side. While his defense team was focused on her, John Murano's head was down, as if watching his cuffed hands squeezed between his knees. The prisoner's slumped back was branded with SUTTER COUNTY JAIL in black letters. To Judge Boleno's left, at the prosecution table, were two young lawyers from the district attorney's office. Vividly animated before the session started, they now had their eyes glued to the judge. They had already won the trial. The only remaining question was how big a feather in their cap this final judgement was going to be.

"We have here also a Court Appointed Special Advocate volunteer for the minor Jack Murano," Judge Boleno continued, nodding to the left of the swing door, in an area separating the officials from the public, where a young boy sat with a middle-aged woman, her arm around his shoulders. He had on gray khaki slacks and a blue polo shirt. His blond hair was neatly slicked. The boy kept shifting his gaze from the woman in the black robe to the man in the orange suit. His hands firmly gripped the bench, as if trying to prevent himself from jumping out of his seat. The CASA official's comforting arm helped him maintain composure in the court of law.

"The defendant was convicted in the deaths of his wife and two people from the other car in an auto accident at the junction of Highways 99 and 20. Mr. Murano was found to be under the influence of alcohol, with a blood level twice the accepted limit. The aggravating circumstances included two previous DUI convictions, with suspensions of license. Additionally, he endangered the life of his then five-year-old son, who was in the vehicle when the accident occurred."

Judge Boleno looked around her courtroom, as if making sure everybody understood the gravity of the defendant's crime.

"The jury," she continued, pointing to the now empty

box, "found the defendant guilty of three counts of Vehicle Code Section 23153--DUI causing injury, and three counts of Penal Code 191.5, gross vehicular manslaughter while intoxicated."

She paused, then stated, "Before the court imposes the sentence, I will call on the attorneys for the district and for the defense. Is there anything you want to state in the court today?"

The defendant raised his head and looked to his lead attorney. The lawyer looked back, then turned to the Judge.

"None for the defense, Your Honor."

Then Judge Boleno looked at the prosecution table.

"None for the prosecution, Your Honor," the young woman from the DA's office said.

Judge Boleno nodded.

"All right. Mr. Murano, if you would, please come around here with your attorney and sit in the witness box."

The defendant hesitated, then got up from his seat and slowly walked to the box with his attorney in tow. He sat in the chair, head down, and looked at his bound wrists, as if in prayer. Then Mr. Murano looked at his son, glued to the CASA volunteer, the boy's eyes piercing him, as if trying to understand the somberness of the proceedings and all that was happening to him since the day his mother died.

"Mr. Murano, you have the right to address the court this morning, prior to the imposition of the sentence. You are not required to say anything, should that be your choice, but the law does afford you that right and opportunity. Is there anything you wish to state to the court this afternoon?"

The defendant stood up and looked at the judge.

"Defendant is not required to stand, Mr. Murano," Judge Boleno said.

"Thank you, Your Honor. I feel better standing," he said.

Then he turned to the boy behind the rail. The prisoner's hair, once black, had been shaved when he was jailed a year ago and was now a mottle of salt-and-pepper stubble. His face looked wrinkled and tired. Only his eyes showed fire. The boy kept staring at him, as if having difficulty recognizing his father.

Murano turned back toward the judge. "Your Honor, I accept full responsibility for what I have done. My wife is dead, and I want to take this last opportunity to apologize to the family of the two people I killed." He stopped and swallowed.

"I'm ready to take any punishment the court will impose on me." His voice broke and he stopped for a few seconds to compose himself. Then he looked at the judge.

"At this moment my single concern is the future of my son. My only hope is that Jack will grow up to be a decent man. He's my only link to the world, and now I won't have any say in his upbringing." He stopped again and looked at his wrists.

"Again, I want to beg the court to make sure my son will be taken care of. That's all. Thank you, Your Honor."

Having said this, Mr. Murano left the witness stand with his lawyer.

"Thank you, sir," Judge Boleno said with a little hesitation. Is he pitying himself? she thought. He had no right to ask for anything. Then she looked at the young boy, who was now piercing her with his big eyes. Judge Boleno knew this look. It took her back to a time in her own life. It was the same look her son had given her when she'd let go of his hand as his stretcher was rolled away to the operating room. He, too, was six at that time. He'd needed surgery to fix his heart defect. Back then, pediatric heart surgery was in its inception, and results were dismal. Many kids did not live through the surgery. She'd known this, but after many hours of painful back-and-forth, she and her husband had decided to proceed. She'd cried throughout the entire seven hours of surgery, until the moment when the doctor came out and informed them that their little boy had survived. Her son was a grown-up man now, but, she thought, he'd had the luxury of both parents helping him during his formative years.

Her mind returning to the moment at hand, Judge Boleno cleared her throat and nodded at Mr. Murano. "Thank you, sir," she repeated.

"Since the jury found you guilty on all counts, the court will not be suspending imposition of sentence. Instead, sentence will be imposed as follows: The sentencing triad for gross vehicular manslaughter while intoxicated is four, six or ten years. As I previously stated, I find that there are aggravating circumstances which support the highest term of ten years in each case. Those circumstances include, but are not limited to, the fact that the defendant has two previous convictions for driving under the influence, there were multiple victims who died in this accident, the defendant's blood alcohol level was more than twice the legal limit, and at the time of the accident, his young son was a passenger in the car."

She rested and looked around the room.

"Therefore, after reviewing all the evidence, and using my best judgement, I impose a total sentence of thirty years in state prison, with nine years to run concurrently thereto."

The courtroom was painfully quiet. The boy looked at his companion, as if asking what all that meant. She just hugged him and shook her head.

"Mr. Murano, you have the right to appeal the judgement the court just entered. If you do appeal, you must do so in writing within sixty days of today's date. If you wish to have an attorney assist you in processing such an appeal, and you cannot afford to hire one, an attorney will be provided for you at no cost. Do you understand? Do you have any questions?"

The defendant looked at his lawyer, who raised his brow slightly. Murano barely shook his head.

"No questions, Your Honor." The lawyer put his hand on the defendant's shoulder.

Judge Boleno started to gather her papers. "Court will stand adjourned."

The bailiff then came to the defense table and stood next to the prisoner. Murano got up slowly, hesitated for a moment, then started to walk towards the exit. Just before the door, he stopped and turned around.

"Daddy!" The boy's voice tore through the still air of the court. Standing with both hands on the railing, the boy tilted forward, as if ready to jump over it. Tears ran down both his cheeks.

The prisoner looked at his son with an expression of unspeakable grief. Then he turned around and disappeared behind the mahogany door.

"SHHIT!" Jack realized he'd missed the exit and had to make a U-turn at the next one.

His mind returned to today's case, and on what could go wrong with the operation. It was going to be a tough one. No question about that.

In the doctor's' lounge, he took a cup of coffee and a doughnut to start his OR day. He changed into scrubs and grabbed another doughnut. He paused to compose himself.

Jack wanted to see Mr. Holden's family one last time before their patriarch was wheeled to room 5. The OR waiting area was just across the hall.

A volunteer directed him to the small conference room––Jack wanted to have more privacy for this crucial conversation with the family. And here they were. Mrs. Holden and her two grown children sat in simple, wooden chairs around the small table, and the volunteer brought a stool for Jack. The son nervously got up seeing Jack entering the room. Did they know about the disaster with Jack's last case? Their faces were somber. Mrs. Holden introduced her children. "They're from out of town," she said. Jack saw the daughter holding her mother's hand, and the son standing next to her, shifting his weight from one leg to the other.

"I want once more to explain Mr. Holden's condition," Jack began. "His heart is damaged and that's the reason for surgery. Dr. Kaplan, his cardiologist, didn't feel comfortable treating him only with medications. He felt that surgery is his last resort. In deciding to take him into the operating room, I am well aware of all the risks he is facing. But it is his only hope, and I promise I will do everything in my power to get him through the surgery and on the way to recovery. I will be with him the entire time and will use all my skills. I just need you to understand all the circumstances."

*I hope I don't sound despondent*, Jack thought as he spoke to the family. But if something were to go wrong, God forbid, and they were to sue, they couldn't say he'd painted a rosy picture. And in his present state of mind, Jack felt anything could happen.

"Do you have any questions?"

Mrs. Holden had teary eyes, both children were looking at her.

"No more questions, doctor," Mrs. Holden said. "My friend is a past patient of yours and has nothing but good things to say about you."

Jack felt a squeeze in his throat. He nodded. Then he left.

On the way to the doctors' lounge, he stopped in the holding room to say hello to Mr. Holden. There his patient lay on a gurney, his arms at his sides, gazing up at the ceiling. A blue, mushroom-like surgical bonnet covered his head and flopped over his left eye, giving him an almost comical look, not fitting the grave situation he was in. Mr. Holden was all by himself. The holding room was empty because heart surgeries were usually performed first, well before the crowds of patients undergoing other operations were brought in. Mr. Holden looked lonely and abandoned. *I know how he feels*, he thought. *Now it's just him and me*.

"Good morning, Mr. Holden. Did you have a good night?" Probably not the best question to start with.

The patient turned his head and smiled. "Tried to. Did you?"

"Yes, I did. No problems." *You don't want to know,* Jack thought. "Do you have any questions, Mr. Holden?"

The patient looked back up at the ceiling for a few seconds, then straight into Jack's eyes.

"Only one, doctor." A pause. "Am I going to wake up?"

Jack's heart stopped. It was the last question he wanted to hear. He took his patient's dried-out, trembling hand in his left hand, then put his right hand on Mr. Holden's forehead and gently stroked it down into the pillow.

"I have not the slightest doubt, Mr. Holden," he lied without blinking his eyes. "No doubts." Then Jack told the truth. "I will do everything in my power to get you through this surgery."

The patient smiled. "I thought so. I trust you."

"Thank you, Mr. Holden."

Jack stroked his forehead again, waited a second, then left the holding area.

In the lounge, Jack drank another two cups of coffee. The other surgeons came in one by one. In cheerful, wound-up voices, they commented on their plans for the upcoming weekend.

Jack didn't want to talk to anybody. He sat in the corner club chair and silently prayed to be able to overcome every foreseen or unforeseen difficulty that could arise during Holden's case.

He was on his own. Yes, he'd have his operating team, but the critical life-and-death decisions would be all his.

"Dr. Murano, you're needed in room 5," the muffled intercom announced.

OR 5 was Jack's dedicated heart room. He opened the swinging door and heard Pavarotti singing "Nessun Dorma." How appropriate, Jack thought. "None shall sleep." Jack hadn't slept before surgery; he wouldn't sleep after. Not until the patient went home. Neither would Mr. Holden's family. The only person able to sleep today would be the patient, on whom anesthesia was working in that very moment. Jack was sure Mr. Holden hadn't slept the night before, and his sleep in the ICU would be frequently interrupted. If he ever gets there. In the opera, Calaf sang, "*Vincero!*" but at that moment Jack felt anything but likely to win. He shook his head.

Jack looked around the room at all the familiar and reassuring faces. Except for one. Next to the anesthesia machine he saw Dr. Matthew Brady, his eyes visible in a slit between the blue surgical cap and green mask. Jack wasn't as comfortable working with Matt on the big cases as he was with Mark Burrow, who was in his opinion the best anesthesiologist around. With Mark Burrow giving anesthesia, Jack didn't have to worry about what was happening on the other side of the ether screen. He didn't have to watch the patient's blood pressure or EKG monitor. Whenever something went wrong, Mark would notify Jack immediately. And with Mark, things seldom went wrong. Jack had requested Mark, but he was already assigned to another case and the OR scheduler couldn't make a change. Matthew Brady would have to do.

It had only been five years since Matt had completed his fellowship, and, in Jack's opinion, he did not have enough experience to handle complex cases. Jack remembered one surgery several months ago when Matt put the patient to sleep for a double valve replacement. During the preparation for cannulation of the heart, while Jack casually talked with his assistant, he suddenly heard Matt's hushed voice from behind the screen: "I have no blood pressure, Jack."

"And you are just telling me this now?" Jack had yelled. His patient was crashing.

"Sorry, Jack," the young man apologized as if he had just stepped on Jack's toe.

*Am I intimidating this guy?* Jack thought.

Jack had to hurry, inserting tubes into the heart and putting the patient on a bypass machine. He'd completed the entire surgery not knowing if the patient would wake up as a vegetable. If the time during which the patient has no blood pressure and no blood flow to the brain is too long, the patient will wake up brain dead. Despite all this, the patient survived and did well.

But Jack's personal acrimony toward Matt hadn't started during that one case. It went back five years earlier, to the day Matt first came to the hospital for a job interview. He had driven to the interview in an old truck and parked diagonally in a spot reserved for the chief of medical staff, taking two spaces. Jack had just recently been elected to that position. He'd fought for that honor for quite a while and saw this perk as one of his proudest accomplishments. The title came with a special parking sign, which, Jack was sure, the new kid must have seen. From the window, Jack had seen his hard-fought-for parking spot hosting an old, beat-up truck that looked as if it had just broken down. Jack had called his auto-mechanic to see what was going on and to get it fixed.

"And please tow this damned thing out of my parking place," he'd added.

Later, clueless, Matt had thanked Jack for helping him out. And today he would be parked on the other side of the screen managing life support during one of Jack's most difficult surgeries.

"We're not ready for you to scrub yet, but Dr. Brady requested that you be here during induction," Cora whispered into Jack's ear. He looked at her—she was rolling her eyes. The beginning of anesthesia on a sick patient could be tricky and Matt obviously wanted Jack to be present in case of trouble.

It took a long time for Matt to put in all the arterial and venous access lines, and that gave Jack time to take a break and have another cup of coffee in the surgeons' lounge.

*I wouldn't have these delays with Mark*, he thought.

A half-hour later, Jack was at the sink, scrubbing. This was his usual time to calm his mind and prepare himself mentally for the procedure. Three minutes with just a hum of running water was enough to put Jack in the proper mood.

He started the operation with the help of Jay, the physician assistant. Jay began his work to take a vein from the patient's leg, to be used to bypass coronary plaques. During the same time, Jack prepared the patient's heart to be connected to the cardiopulmonary bypass machine.

Then the wall phone rang.

"Dr. Stone is here," Cora said, holding the receiver to her chest. "Should we ask him to scrub?" Dan Stone was Jack's partner, whom he had asked for help on this complicated case.

"A few more minutes. We just gave heparin," Jack answered. Holden's blood had to be thinned so it would not clot in the tubings. Jay had harvested the vein and already closed the leg incision.

Jack watched the patient's exposed heart. With the thick layer of fat on the surface, it contracted slowly, deliberately, having great difficulty pushing blood through the diseased valve. Jack could feel the surgical cap already wet on his forehead.

"I want to have a balloon in the room," he said.

The intra-aortic balloon pump is a device used when a sick patient cannot be weaned off pump support. It's reserved for dire situations. At the very least, in Jack's experience and that of his team, it meant long hours in OR 5.

Cora, the circulating nurse, left the room and promptly came back wheeling a small console that powered the heart-assist device. Everybody in the room got quiet.

Dan Stone came in and, seeing the balloon console at the end of the operating table, raised his eyebrows at Cora. She nodded.

By this time, the boombox was playing the second part of Paganini's fourth violin concerto. A lovely cantilena. Jack had always thought that if this piece didn't move you, nothing would. But not so today.

"Stop the music," he snapped. "I want to have complete quiet through the rest of this case."

The only sound they could hear now was the beeping of the heart monitor.

Jack and Dan worked around the heart. No one talked. Cora took the wall phone's receiver off the hook and put it down on the little table standing right below.

They went on the bypass and stopped the heart. Jack knew that now time was critical. Even with the best preservation techniques, Mr. Holden's weak heart couldn't be arrested for long. They had to do all the necessary work within the shortest possible time. No coffee breaks allowed.

They hooked the veins to the coronary arteries first. Nothing unexpected happened. Jack always thought that if he was the best surgeon in the hospital, Dan was certainly the best assistant. Together, they were a great team. Their hands moved in unison, as if connected with invisible strings.

Next, Jack excised the old, diseased valve. Joni handed him a sizer.

"Number 22, homograft." He wanted to use a human biological valve, as opposed to a mechanical, man-made. He wanted to spare the patient life-long need for blood thinners.

No problems so far. Two surgeons working flawlessly together, anticipating each other's needs. Watching Jack's hands, one could see occasional tremors, and his movements were becoming hurried. He kept looking at the clock.

Joni, his best scrub nurse, had known him for years and was starting to worry. Jack Murano, she knew, was completely silent only under immense pressure. She leaned over to him.

"Dr. Murano," she whispered. "Relax." She saw him watching the clock.

"I'm fine," Jack responded. But he wasn't, and Joni knew it.

A minute later: "Dr. Murano, you're doing great. Time to slow down." Only Joni could talk to him that way.

"I'm fine," he barked, stopping in the middle of the stitch and giving her a stern look.

No more comments.

After replacing the valve, the two surgeons attached the veins to the aorta above. It took time, despite both surgeons working precisely together.

Jack again looked at the clock. The length of time Holden's heart had been stopped was long, but Jack was doing his best to protect the muscle with proper cold solution injected into the coronary circulation and ice slush around it.

Finally, they finished all work with the heart. Now it was time to warm up the patient and wean him off the support. The machine had to be disconnected, and the heart, after having been stopped, had to start beating on its own again and take over. Every time Jack saw this happen in the OR, he felt he was witnessing a miracle.

He kept checking the clock. Mr. Holden's heart hadn't beaten in more than two hours. Way longer than he had wanted.

For this part, Jack didn't need an assistant—now he could work by himself. Besides, he didn't want his partner around any longer.

"Dan, I think I'll be okay now," he said. "Thanks for coming."

"Are you sure?" Dan hesitated. "I'll be in the doctor's lounge. Just in case."

Jack knew his partner sensed that anything could go wrong at any moment.

"Thanks again, Dan," he said.

Jack felt mentally drained. His cap felt wet, and he could see and feel the slime under his gloves.

He was on his own again.

"Are we warm enough?"

"Yes, thirty-six degrees," Ron at the pump said. He was clearly in control of his job. The hypothermia was reversed, and the time had come for Mr. Holden's heart to take over.

"Ready to come off?"

"Ready when you are. Here we go."

Jack clamped the large tube draining the heart and saw its muscle slowly filling up with the blood still coming from the pump. He watched his patient gradually taking over from the machine. He knew he had done the procedure flawlessly. Despite having a sense of accomplishment, however, Jack felt uneasy. Now came the real-life test. Would Holden's repaired heart beat well on its own?

"Are you ready?" Jack asked Matt.

"Yep, we are ready," he answered.

They gradually slowed the machine support down, but the miraculous blob of the heart muscle, usually slightly bigger than a fist, suddenly got twice as big, contracted sluggishly, lazily, and was unable to pump its blood. Holden's heart was failing. After watching the organ struggle for several minutes, Jack ordered, "Let's go back on the bypass. Let him rest. And max all the drips."

*Why do I have to tell him what to do?* Jack thought, looking at Matt.

The room was dead quiet. Everybody concentrated on their jobs. Ron, with a tube clamp in his hand, adjusted the speed of the pump, reading Jack the flow numbers on the monitor. Joni, the scrub nurse, kept moving the instruments on her table, trying to anticipate Jack's next request. Cora, the circulating nurse, concentrated on the blood pressure and EKG monitors. Only Matt Brady and his nurse anesthetist were in constant motion, responding instantly to changes in blood pressure, heart rate, and the patient's oxygen level. They had to manipulate the infusion rate of medications regulating heart function. They kept checking the potassium level. They watched how much urine was in the bag. They measured the oxygen level. And they constantly watched the EKG monitor and blood pressure readouts.

Seeing Matt in constant motion, Jack remained still. But there was turmoil in his head. *Why is Matt so busy?* He thought. *Does he know what he's doing? How I wish Mark was here.*

"Dr. Murano, do you need a stool?" Cora whispered from behind him.

Jack didn't even turn around. He just shook his head. He felt dizzy. She put the stool next to him just in case.

The pump now worked at full speed, giving Mr. Holden's tired heart muscle time to rest and replenish its meager energy reserves.

Jack waited another fifteen minutes and again tried to wean him off machine support. Again, the heart pumped for a while, then it got distended, started to contract lazily, and failed. Jack felt heat and pulsations in his head. His hands were shaking. He remembered the last time he'd had these feelings. It was a few years ago. His patient's heart couldn't take over after multiple trials, and eventually machine support had to be stopped. The patient had died. The worst part was the heartbreaking conversation with the family afterward, telling them that their father had not survived the surgery. He still cringed whenever he thought of that case.

Now Jack sat on the stool.

Mr. Holden seemed headed in the same direction. The likelihood that his heart would take over the workload from the machine diminished every minute.

*He can't handle it*, Jack thought, looking at Matt.

The pulsations in Jack's head got stronger. He felt as if a big kettledrum was beating hard, becoming louder and faster every minute. Jack jumped up.

"Get me the balloon!" he yelled, stomping his foot twice. The nurses in the room looked at each other. Nothing like this had ever happened in Dr. Murano's operating room before.

Cora quickly opened a long plastic container with a flexible rod and a long, narrow, inflatable balloon wrapped around its end.

"Introducer!" Joni said, handing Jack a plastic sheath that he swiftly put into the artery in the patient's groin.

"Stitch!" He fixed the sheath to the skin.

They went back on the bypass. Mr. Holden's heart still had no strength to take over.

Now Jack's actions resembled those of an enraged tiger locked in a cage—in his case, OR 5, where he was confined with five others—and the walls amplified his rage.

"Do you want me to call Dr. Stone back?" Cora came behind him and whispered.

"I'll be fine," Jack snarled. He got up from the stool and started pacing around the table. He didn't want the drama of Stone being called back to alert the rest of the operating block staff to his problems. Soon he would have the entire OR peeking through the windows. He couldn't take any more personal setbacks.

The counter-pulsations of the balloon became synchronized with the external pacemaker, and Jack tried to get Mr. Holden off the bypass machine again. Finally, slowly, with the incremental withdrawal of the pump support, with the coordinated help of the intra-aortic balloon, and with the full doses of medications being given by Matt, the patient was weaned off the machine and his heart began beating on its own.

Jack left all the tubes in, just in case. Each heartbeat was stimulated by the wires attached to the external pacemaker and synchronized with the pulsations of the intra-aortic balloon. Everybody and everything were working at maximal effort. Still, the patient's heart looked as if it was working the hardest, at the very limits of its capacity.

It struggled.

And struggled.

Jack felt hot, despite the room's cool temperature. His own heart seemed to be jumping up to his neck. He felt hot and sweaty, while all the other people in the operating room had warming blankets on their shoulders.

"Let's wait before we close." Jack had reached the limits of his tolerance. He was sitting on the stool again, his eyes fixated on the EKG monitor and the blood pressure numbers. Too many extra beats, he thought. Not what he wanted to see. But Mr. Holden's pressure numbers were still acceptable.

The operating room was quiet––no music, no one took breaks. Anything could happen anytime now. Everybody knew that. Was Mr. Holden going to make it, or was this the calm before the storm? Jack waited another fifteen minutes, then, with Jay's help, he removed the cannulas from the heart. First venous, then aortic. He sat on his stool, waiting, and waiting, with Mr. Holden's chest still open. The heart monitor kept showing many extra beats. Not a good sign. He was aware that many extra beats could signal severe, often fatal heart arrhythmias. Mr. Holden's blood pressure held steady without the help of the bypass machine but was on the low side. Not much bleeding, though. This encouraged Jack. Still, he didn't want to commit himself to closing the chest. Not yet. If Mr. Holden crashed and needed to go back on the pump support, valuable time would be lost in having to open his chest again. Everyone in the OR waited silently.

Then, out of the blue, the EKG monitor showed a high zigzag burst of heart fibrillation. It looked like an earthquake on a seismograph.

Jack jumped up from his stool.

"Charge the paddles!" he yelled.

Matt reached toward the defibrillator box.

"Pacer off!" Jack commanded.

Matt turned off the pacemaker.

It took two shocks to stop fibrillation, but the shocks also stopped the heart. The EKG monitor showed a straight line.

"Pacer on!" Matt Brady was working furiously behind the anesthesia screen.

"Max the drips!" But the patient's blood pressure was barely detectable.

*What is he doing?* Jack's brain recoiled as he watched Matt. *Why can't he handle this case? I wish Mark was here. Why did I agree to have Matt put this patient to sleep?*

Jack felt as if his head was going to explode. *I am going to lose him*! Those words screamed in Jack's head. Somehow, he mustered enough willpower to control himself.

Then, after another burst of ventricular fibrillation and after another shock, Mr. Holden's blood pressure fell to zero.

"Back on bypass!" Jack yelled.

This was a daunting task because all the tubes

connecting the patient's heart to the cardiopulmonary bypass machine were out. Jack had to again put one cannula into the aorta and another large bore drain into his big vein. This took a few minutes, and meanwhile Holden's brain had no blood flow. If it took longer than five minutes, the patient could end up with a brain death.

"Stitch!" Jack screamed to the scrub nurse.

"Not that, aortic!"

Jack looked at the needle holder Joni gave him and threw it across the room. The scrub dropped her head. She had never seen Murano in such an emotional mess.

With trembling hands, and without a second to spare, he connected his patient to the machine again. Jack wanted to give his patient's heart some rest and then let it try to take over again. But this was not happening. *They're watching me*, he thought. *I can't give up. Never, never.* Jack looked around and saw all the eyes on him. He couldn't quit now.

But nothing Jack did seemed to change the inevitable.

Mr. Holden was dying.

Now Jack didn't even have to even look around and see their eyes. He could feel them watching his every move. He knew they were watching him trying so hard not to let the patient go. But he'd failed them. Jack became quiet and he slumped onto the stool.

*My patient is dead.* The words shot through Jack's mind. *I can't get him off the bypass. There's nothing else I can do to save him.*

He got up, slowly went around the table, and stood in front of Matt Brady.

"You killed this patient!" Jack yelled, pointing his finger at Matt's chest. The younger man's eyes, visible between his surgical cap and his mask, grew round, his head shook back, and his entire body jerked. Then Matt's eyebrows frowned, but he didn't utter a word. He just looked at Jack.

In his own mind, Jack felt he couldn't fall any lower.

~

JACK SLOWLY TURNED AROUND. He looked as if someone had let the air out of his silhouette. Slouching, he staggered to the corner of the room. He methodically removed his gown, gloves, and mask, threw them on the ground, and left the operating room.

The room became as quiet as intergalactic space. All heads were lowered. Joni shuffled instruments on her tray. Ron continued filling out the pump sheets. Cora stood brushing invisible specs from her scrubs. Matt Brady looked white, stunned, bewildered by what had just happened. They were all stunned.

JACK WALKED to the lounge and poured himself a cup of coffee. There he sat, his hands shaking and his head pulsating. Two surgeons sitting nearby momentarily stopped talking and looked at him. *They already know*, Jack thought. *Word spreads fast in this damned place.*

The prospect of talking to the Holden family sickened him. How was he going to tell them? He knew of no way to explain what had just happened, no way to express his desolation. Jack needed to gather himself while he came up with some kind of strategy. He'd wait for a few minutes. Half an hour?

He called the front desk and asked the charge nurse to tell the Holdens that the patient was not doing well.

How could he console the family? He sat in the corner

chair and rested his head in both hands. He needed some time before asking the charge nurse to gather Holden's family in the conference room.

What was he going to say to them? He felt guilty, despite having told them before surgery that anything could happen.

Then he thought of other consequences. Would the executive committee sanction him? Would they impose a mandatory proctor for his future cases? Would they put him on probation?

He leaned back in his chair, stretched his legs, and closed his eyes. Both hands landed on his chest.

Then, suddenly, the voice from the intercom shook him again, like a jolt from a defibrillator.

"Dr. Murano, you are needed in room 5, stat! Dr. Murano . . ."

*What now? What could they possibly need me for now in this miserable place? It's too soon to pronounce the patient dead. That can be done later. They still have to remove the tubes, IVs, and catheters and cover the body with a white sheet. What in the world?*

Jack jumped out of his seat and ran back to his operating room.

The place was quiet. He looked at his team and saw everyone moving methodically. Joni covered the open chest with a sterile towel. Cora assisted Dr. Brady with getting and connecting the IV bags and injecting the medications through the piggyback ports. Ron stood by the blood gas machine checking the most recent sample. Matt calmly directed the team, asking questions and, in a composed voice, giving them orders.

The room looked peaceful. It was a scene from another world.

Jack looked at the monitor. It showed a blood pressure of 100 and an EKG showing a heart rhythm properly paced by an external pacemaker.

His patient was alive!

What the hell had happened?

The unbelievable had occurred. And yet, he'd heard stories like this in the past. Now Jack felt embarrassed and humiliated. His team had brought the patient back while he was drinking coffee in the lounge, having given up. And mourning *his* misfortune.

He looked at his crew. No one even noticed him. They were all busy working. Jack didn't belong there. Matt Brady was in charge. With the help of his nurse anesthetist, he was infusing residual blood from the pump into Mr. Holden while Ron stood by the machine checking the latest potassium levels. Joni helped Jay stop small bleeders from the patient's chest wall, and Cora was on the phone, ordering medications from the OR pharmacy.

Jack felt like a slashed tire as he stood there watching.

Would they even want to work with him again? Would he ever be able to regain their trust? His head felt as if it was ready to explode.

Jack scrubbed at the outside sink and rejoined his team. In dead silence he finished the operation and closed Mr. Holden's chest himself. Then he stood up in the middle of the room and said what he knew he needed to say.

"I am really sorry for my behavior today. This has never happened to me in the past and it will never happen in the future. You guys did a magnificent job, and I will never be able to repay you for that. Again, I am very, very sorry."

Jack was speaking to everyone, but he was looking at Matt.

Then he left the room.

After a few minutes he asked the nurses to gather Holden's family in a conference room—the same room where he had explained the perils of the upcoming surgery that morning.

He entered and once again all eyes turned to him. By closing the door behind him, he was isolating himself from the noise of the adjacent, now-busy OR waiting room. He wanted to separate himself from the events of the last several hours, which seemed like forever ago. The cramped conference room was as quiet as the operating room he'd just left.

Jack took a seat and a few seconds to compose himself.

"I have good news for you," he said. "Mr. Holden is doing fine. The surgery went well, although not without difficulties. We replaced a valve and bypassed the blockages in his coronaries. His heart was weak, and we had to insert an aortic balloon to temporarily assist its work. But he's okay now and off the bypass machine."

"Any problems?" Mr. Holden's son asked.

"Nothing that we couldn't resolve," Jack replied, momentarily looking at the floor. "I had the best team available for your father's surgery today," he added.

"When will we be able to see him?"

"Within an hour or so. The ICU nurse will let you know. He is still in the operating room."

"Thank you, Dr. Murano," the daughter said. She had tears in her eyes. Mrs. Holden just kept looking at him.

*She doesn't believe me*, Jack thought.

The son seemed relieved.

LEAVING THE FAMILY, Jack lumbered into the empty surgeons' lounge. He turned off the TV and collapsed into the cushy chair. He felt pounding in his head and his hands shook. He wanted to get out of the hospital to some secluded, quiet beach. All by himself. Just out of this damned place.

Matt Brady! How had he brought the patient back?

"Never give up!" That was Jack's line. He lived by it. He always tried to chisel it into his kids' minds. But it only counts when you remember it and follow it in the proper time. That morning he'd been tired, lifeless. He'd expected defeat from the beginning. The exhaustion and fear had made him a coward. When Jack was at the bottom, Matt stepped up, and this after being blamed for the disaster!

Just then, the lounge door opened and in walked Matt Brady.

Jack had not expected this meeting so soon after the case. Not knowing what to do, he stood up, ready to leave if it came to a confrontation.

Matt had a bleak smile on his face and Jack didn't know if it was a friendly or a triumphant smile. He had to be prepared for both.

"Matt," he said, "I am truly sorry for my behavior during this case. I have a lot on my mind and didn't handle the pressure well. I had no reason to blame it on you. I will be forever grateful to you for bringing this patient back."

The anesthesiologist didn't seem to be in a hurry. He poured a cup of coffee and sat at the low table.

"Jack," he finally said, "let me tell you a story. You may even remember it." He took a sip of coffee and his eyes drifted upward, above Jack's head.

"The first time I visited this hospital was five or so years ago. It was at the end of my fellowship, and I came here for a job interview. It wasn't my only interview; I had a few more places to visit before deciding where to start my practice.

"When I came here, my old truck broke down in the hospital parking lot and I was stuck. I had several appointments set up, here and at other offices in town, with no means of getting to them. You were leaving the hospital at the time and saw me meditating under the lifted hood. Do you remember?"

Jack furrowed his brow, pretending he was digging in his memory. Of course, he did!

"You called your mechanic and had him fix it. The damage was so bad he had to tow it to the shop."

Jack dropped his head and showed a despondent smile. "I remember. You looked a little lost," Jack said softly.

"I felt horrible." Matt continued. "I'd come so far and then *that*."

"My interviews went fine. I got a job offer from this hospital, as well as a few others. Finally, I had to make a choice."

Matt stopped and stretched his legs.

"I chose this hospital. Do you know why?" He leaned over and rested his elbows on the table.

"I came here because of you. If people like you worked here, I thought, I wanted to be part of that culture."

Jack felt a spasm in his throat and his vision blurred. He knew not to look at Matt's face. He nodded, but kept his head bowed low. The man he hadn't respected from the beginning, whom he had regarded begrudgingly all these years for parking in his damn parking space, had proved himself beyond all expectations, and not only saved his patient's life but also Jack's reputation.

He looked at Matt and said quietly, "Thank you."

Dr. Brady thought for a while, as if debating what to say next.

'There's another thing," he continued. "After meeting you in the parking lot, I went to the OR to introduce myself to the chief of anesthesia and to have a tour of the department. A couple of nurses stopped and started talking to me. They'd seen the two of us standing next to my dilapidated truck and asked if you were my father. We looked alike, they said."

It was totally quiet in the room. Jack couldn't even look into Matt's eyes.

"You know, Jack, I grew up without my father. He left us when I was ten years old. I never saw him again. I missed terribly all the activities I saw my childhood friends having with their fathers. Then, from the time we met here, I felt this unusual bond with you, wishing my father, who I barely knew, was still around. Meeting you felt like having found that missing piece of my life puzzle. You came and filled up the void in my life."

Matt stopped, then added. "I won't let that happen to my son. I hope to be a better father to him than my father was to me."

Jack got up, bent over, and gave Matt a hug. It was longer than just a casual embrace.

In that moment, Jack felt as if he was hugging himself.

## ABOUT THE AUTHOR

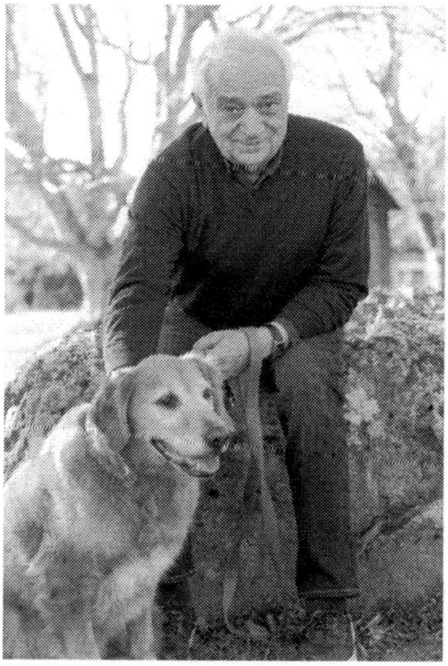

*With Bentley*

After a thirty-plus career as a cardiac surgeon in California, I decided to retire and moved to Chapel Hill, North Carolina, where I live now with my wife Bonnie and golden retriever Bentley. Following many years spent in the operating room, I discovered my new passion––writing. It took me a long time to collect all the stories, but it was worth it. Half of the stories I write about are the truth, but no one knows which half.

# BEFORE YOU GO

Throughout my life, I've been wearing many hats. It's like riding the waves. First, I was a student in my school in a lovely part of Warsaw, Żoliborz. In the morning I got my classical education under the watchful eye of Mrs. Libera, who taught Latin, ancient history, and, after hours, French. In the afternoon, my mother was bringing my violin, and it was time for music education. Mrs. Zawadzka made sure my technique was improving, and Mr. Kolasiński expanded my horizon with history and theory of music. I graduated from both schools with honors. Then I started my medical education in Warsaw Medical School. When there, I also wore a second hat. It was my memorable stint with volleyball. With my friends, I was privileged to win the national championship. Twice.

The medical hat, acquired in Poland, I carried to the United States. Here it got a cardiac surgical badge and lasted through my second trimester of my life.

But I wasn't meant to be a surgeon for life. For the third trimester, I chose the career of a writer. I couldn't dream of better passion in my retirement. People ask me why I waited so long. I tell them it took me that long to gather all the materials.

It looks like that's my final hat.

# KEEP IN TOUCH

Dear Reader,

You went that far in reading this book, and I am grateful for your effort. Without the exaggeration, I feel honored. For a writer, the fact of a reader spending time with his work is a bliss. Again, thanks.

If you're willing to visit my website—here it is.

If you wish to read my blog—here is the link.

You are welcome to subscribe on the website.

Made in the USA
Monee, IL
13 September 2026

62979555R00028